WEIGHT GAIN DIET BOOK

Maximize Muscle Growth, Enhance Athletic Performance, Boost Metabolism, and Strengthen Immunity for Optimal Stamina and Overall Health

Audrey McAllister, MD

Copyright Page

laws and regulations. By accessing or using any part of this work, individuals agree to comply with the terms and conditions set forth by the publisher regarding copyright protection and usage rights.

Table of Contents

SECTION I: UNDERSTANDING WEIGHT GAIN

Weight gain is when your weight increases due to changes in your body composition, like increased fat, muscle, or fluids. It is normal for people to experience weight changes throughout different stages of life, including puberty, pregnancy, and aging. Consult with your healthcare provider if you're concerned about weight gain.

Factors Contributing to Difficulty in Gaining Weight

High Metabolism

One of the primary challenges faced by individuals trying to gain weight is having a high metabolism.

Metabolism refers to the rate at which your body burns calories. Individuals with a high metabolism tend to burn calories quickly, making it difficult for them to gain weight. Increasing calorie intake may be necessary to counterbalance the fast metabolism and achieve weight gain.

Poor Appetite

Another challenge is having a poor appetite. Some individuals naturally have a small appetite or struggle to eat large quantities of food. This can make it challenging to consume a sufficient amount of calories needed for weight gain. It is important to find strategies to increase appetite, such as eating smaller, more frequent meals, incorporating calorie-dense foods, and including snacks throughout the day.

Dietary Restrictions or Preferences

Dietary restrictions or preferences can also pose challenges when trying to gain weight. For example, individuals following a vegetarian or vegan diet may find it more difficult to consume enough protein, which is crucial for muscle growth and weight gain. It is important to carefully plan meals to ensure an adequate intake of all essential nutrients, including protein, carbohydrates, and healthy fats.

Busy Lifestyle

A busy lifestyle can be a significant challenge when trying to gain weight. Individuals who are constantly on the go may find it difficult to prioritize meals or find time to prepare calorie-dense meals. It is essential to plan ahead, carry snacks or meal replacements, and incorporate quick and easy-to-prepare meals into the daily routine to ensure consistent calorie intake.

Psychological Factors

Psychological factors can also influence weight gain. Some individuals may have a negative body image or struggle with disordered eating patterns, which can hinder their ability to gain weight. Addressing these psychological factors through therapy or counseling can be crucial in overcoming the challenges and establishing a healthy relationship with food and body.

Lack of Knowledge and Guidance

A lack of knowledge and guidance on effective weight gain strategies can be a significant challenge for individuals. It is important to seek information from credible sources, consult with healthcare professionals or registered dietitians, and develop a personalized weight gain plan based on individual needs and goals.

For others, underlying medical conditions and certain medical treatments may cause weight loss or difficulty gaining weight. These include the following conditions.

Hyperthyroidism

An overactive thyroid, or hyperthyroidism, causes an excess of thyroid hormone in the body. Thyroid hormone is responsible for many elements of human metabolism, including regulation of metabolic rate.

People with hyperthyroidism have an overactive metabolism and often burn more calories throughout the day. Without the proper medication, hyperthyroidism can cause trouble gaining weight, even when food intake is increased.

Type 1 diabetes

Type 1 diabetes is a type of autoimmune condition in which the body destroys the cells in the pancreas that are responsible for the production of insulin.

Insulin is the hormone responsible for the metabolism of glucose. When type 1 diabetes goes unmanaged, it causes high levels of blood glucose, which is then excreted in the urine. This excess glucose excretion can lead to unintentional weight loss.

Inflammatory bowel disease

Inflammatory bowel disease (IBD) is a blanket term for a series of conditions characterized by inflammation of the intestines. These conditions, such as Crohn's disease and ulcerative colitis, can have negative impacts on someone's ability to maintain weight.

These conditions may limit the types and amounts of food that a person can eat. They may also cause frequent diarrhea, which can cause weight loss in some cases.

Eating disorders

While there are many different types of disordered eating conditions, people with eating disorders that limit food intake may have trouble maintaining a healthy weight.

In its most extreme form, anorexia nervosa causes extreme weight loss and sometimes the inability to gain weight entirely. Other conditions, such as bulimia, can make it hard for a person to keep enough calories down to maintain weight.

Medications and treatments

Certain medications and treatments that cause appetite loss, nausea, vomiting, and diarrhea can make it difficult to maintain a healthy weight.

For example, medications like antibiotics and treatments like chemotherapy are commonly known for causing gastrointestinal side effects.

Generally, people who require these types of treatments may experience weight loss and have difficulty gaining weight throughout treatment.

Importance of a Balanced Approach to Weight Gain

Achieving weight gain in a balanced manner is really important for a few key reasons:

1. Health and Nutrition: It's not just about putting on weight; it's about doing it in a way that benefits your overall health. Balancing your diet and exercise helps ensure you gain muscle along with fat, which is better for your body in the long run.

2. Sustainable Progress: Rushing to gain weight can cause problems later on. Taking a balanced approach allows your body to adjust gradually, making it easier to maintain your new weight once you reach your goal.

3. Physical Performance: When you gain weight through balanced nutrition and exercise, you're not only building muscle but also improving your strength and stamina.

4. Mental Well-being: Rapid weight gain or unhealthy eating habits can affect how you feel about yourself. By taking a balanced approach, you're promoting a healthier relationship with food and your body, which is good for your mental health.

5. Long-term Success: By focusing on balanced nutrition and regular exercise, you're setting yourself up for long-term success. This consistency is key to achieving and keeping a healthy weight.

6. Nutrient Balance: A balanced approach ensures you're getting all the nutrients your body needs. Rapid weight gain from unhealthy foods can lead to deficiencies in important vitamins and minerals.

SECTION II: PLANNING YOUR WEIGHT GAIN DIET

Weight Gain through Diet Patterns

Here are a few ways you can encourage faster weight gain through your diet pattern:

• **Prioritize nutrient-dense foods:** Choose nutrient-dense foods to ensure that essential vitamins and minerals accompany your weight gain. Include fruits, vegetables, lean proteins, whole grains, and healthy fats in your diet.

• **Maintain balance:** A balanced diet includes carbohydrates, proteins, and fats. This helps support overall health and provides the energy necessary for weight gain.

• **Eat regularly:** Be consistent with your meals and include nutritious snacks to maintain a steady calorie intake throughout the day. For example, instead of eating three large meals daily, perhaps you can switch to five slightly smaller meals and three snacks.

• **Opt for larger portion sizes:** Serve yourself more than you usually would, particularly with calorie-dense foods. If you're not hungry for it, don't stuff yourself, but also don't limit yourself if you're interested in eating more than usual in a sitting.

• **Use sauces and dressings:** When you've put together your meal or snack, consider adding healthy toppings and sauces to enhance your meals' flavor and calorie content. Examples of this can include olive oil and vinegar, guacamole, hummus, or a yogurt-based dressing.

Meal Prep for Weight Gain

It is important to prepare meals and snacks ahead of time to successfully gain weight.

First, decide what meals and snacks will be best consumed, focusing on favorite dishes and flavors. It can also be beneficial to take note of in-season foods, so grocery shopping is easier and more wallet-friendly.

Second, make your shopping list by food category. Include: dairy, fruit, vegetables, meat, bread/grains, canned foods, spices, desserts, drinks, etc. This will make the shopping trip quick and easy and will ensure you don't forget any foods.

Third, you can meal prep for the week by batch cooking and chopping vegetables. Batch cooking is cooking large quantities of foods that will be needed throughout the week for multiple meals.

For example, bake/grill a few extra chicken breasts and refrigerate for later use. Remove from the refrigerator and microwave when it is time to serve the meal. Please note that cooked chicken will only keep in the refrigerator for 3-4 days.

Finally, choose a few favorite meals and serve them multiple times a week. This allows for even more batch cooking and for easier shopping trips because there are less ingredients needed.

Weight Gaining Strategies to Apply

Outside of having an underlying medical condition, the truth is that it's more difficult for some people to gain weight than others.

If you're having trouble gaining weight, there are certain lifestyle changes you can make to give yourself the best chance of increasing your body weight in a healthy manner.

Build more muscle

Both cardio and weight training are important for overall health, but weight training is an absolute must when you want to build more muscle.

Since muscle weighs more than fat, weight training can help you increase your overall weight without just increasing your overall body fat.

Eat frequent meals

Eating meals more frequently can allow you to consume more calories throughout the day — especially if you're someone who doesn't enjoy huge meals.

Breaking bigger meals into smaller, more frequent meals can allow you to eat more calories without having to uncomfortably stack your plate or fill your stomach.

Enjoy high calorie foods

Meals high in whole grains and healthy fats tend to have more calories than meals consisting of lower calorie foods, such as lean proteins and vegetables.

Start each meal with at least a cup of grains, and try to incorporate various fats, such as oils, nuts, or other condiments. Finally, finish with some lean protein and at least a few servings of vegetables.

Use more condiments

Condiments, especially those that are high in fat, can add at least a few hundred calories to any meal.

For example, light drizzling oils and mayonnaise-based sauces can help bulk up a sandwich, wrap, or even a salad.

Try shakes and supplements

If you're still struggling to meet your daily calorie goals, protein shakes and supplements can help add extra calories to your daily intake.

Meal replacement shakes tend to be higher in calories and are aimed at maintaining weight for people who can't consume regular food. Also, some protein shakes are formulated specifically for building body mass.

Don't fill up on water

For a lot of people, drinking water before a meal can help them avoid overeating — but this trick can backfire if you're trying to gain weight.

It's still important to drink water frequently throughout the day, but if you're having trouble eating meals because of fullness, avoid drinking too much water before you sit down to your meal.

SECTION III: NUTRITIONAL FOUNDATIONS FOR WEIGHT GAIN

Caloric Surplus: How Many Calories Do You Need?

Increasing your total calorie intake is the best way to gain weight quickly. One common guideline is to aim for a surplus of 500–1,000 calories per day to gain weight at a moderate and sustainable rate. This could lead to a weight gain of about 1 or 2 pounds per week. Remember that these numbers are rough estimates, and individual needs may vary.

Here's a basic approach to determining your daily calorie needs for weight gain:

1. Calculate basal metabolic rate (BMR): Use an online BMR calculator to estimate the calories your body needs at rest.

2. Factor in physical activity: Multiply your BMR by an activity factor representing your daily physical activity level (sedentary, lightly active, moderately active, very active).

3. Add a caloric surplus: Add 500–1,000 calories to the calculated total to gain weight. This is the number of calories you should aim to consume each day.

Of course, boosting your calorie intake isn't the whole story. Considering the details of your overall diet to achieve long-term, sustainable changes to your weight is also important.

Macronutrient Ratios: Carbohydrates, Proteins, and Fats

When it comes to building muscle, the right diet plays a crucial role in achieving your goals. Weight gain, which is essential for muscle growth, is accomplished by consuming a surplus of calories through a well-planned bulking diet. However, it's important to note that muscle growth should be combined with regular physical activity, such as resistance training, to maximize results.

To determine the exact number of calories you should consume, it's important to consider your body type and calculate your caloric needs based on your muscle gain preferences and physical activity levels. To gain muscle, you'll need to enhance your protein intake and adhere to a high-calorie diet. However, you will also need to strike a balance and avoid excessive consumption, as it may lead to undesired gains in body fat. This personalized approach ensures that you are providing your body with the necessary fuel to support muscle growth without excessive calorie intake.

Understanding the right macronutrients (macros) for building muscle is equally important. Protein, the most essential macro for gaining lean mass, should be a cornerstone of your diet. Incorporating lean protein sources, such as chicken, fish, tofu, and legumes, into your weight gain meals helps provide the necessary amino acids for muscle repair and growth.

Carbohydrates, the second vital macro, fuel your workouts by replenishing glycogen stores and supporting muscle recovery. Opt for high-quality carbohydrates like whole grains, fruits, and vegetables, as they provide sustained energy and essential nutrients. Avoid simple carbohydrates that can cause spikes in sugar levels and offer little nutritional value.

Fat, the third essential macro, serves as a source of long-lasting energy. Since fat provides more than twice the calories per gram compared to protein and carbohydrates, it's important to moderate your intake. Consuming too much fat in a calorie surplus can lead to increased fat storage. Choose healthy sources of fats like nuts, seeds, avocados, and olive oil.

Incorporating nutrient-dense fruits and vegetables into your diet is crucial. They not only provide high-quality carbohydrates but also supply essential vitamins, minerals, and antioxidants. Lean proteins, as mentioned earlier, are vital for their amino acid content and should be prioritized in your meals.

By following a well-balanced diet that includes the right balance of macros, quality proteins, and nutrient-dense foods, you can provide your body with the necessary ingredients for muscle growth while supporting overall health. Combine this diet with a consistent exercise routine, and you'll be on your way to achieving your muscle-building goals.

Micronutrients: Essential Vitamins and Minerals for Muscle Growth

1. Vitamin D

Vitamin D is the most important vitamin for bodybuilders when it comes to muscle growth and recovery. Obtaining Vitamin D is unique in that the body or especially your skin needs exposure to direct sunlight to start its production.

Another important function of Vitamin D is to keep diseases away. We know that many people who don't get enough sunlight exposure are deficient, but how can it support muscle growth and recovery?

Well, vitamin D is the most important of all vitamins when it comes to testosterone production. Some research studies even show that vitamin D supplementation can significantly increase explosive power in adults, together with a strength-training program, in comparison to placebo subjects.

Vitamin D even plays a key role in protein synthesis, which is partly due to its impact on testosterone production. In fact, a study conducted on men with low testosterone found that supplementation with vitamin D led to a 20% increase in free testosterone.

In addition to its effects on testosterone and muscle growth, vitamin D can also improve bone health. Vitamin D works alongside calcium and magnesium, which are essential minerals for bone development.

2. Vitamin C

We've all had a common cold and been given advice such as, "Make sure you increase your vitamin C intake," but what about benefits for muscle growth and recovery?

One of the most powerful antioxidants, Vitamin C comes in at No. 2 on the list. When you exercise, you damage muscle tissue, creating free radicals, which are harmful compounds that your body must remove. Antioxidants clean up and destroy free radicals, which benefit your training and enhances your recovery.

Vitamin C is also a tremendous immunity booster, helping to prevent sickness. This is especially beneficial in times of physical stress such as when you are engaging in more intense training or low-carb dieting.

Vitamin C is water-soluble, meaning your body doesn't store it, so you need to ingest it daily in supplement or food form to make sure it's available to optimize physiological function.

Vitamin C Dosage

Take 500-2,000 milligrams per day in supplement form. More than 1,000 milligrams at one time may cause gastrointestinal disturbances, so introduce vitamin C supplementation in small doses if you're not currently taking it.

For best results, start with one 500 milligram dose per day for the first week, and then add 500-milligram dose per day the following week. Continue with this method until you reach 2,000 milligrams or your desired daily dosage.

Best Food Sources for Vitamin C

Orange juice, grapefruit juice, peaches, sweet red capsicums, and papaya.

Whole oranges and grapefruits are also good sources of vitamin C, but their relatively low concentration of calories compared to juice (which contains more sugars, hence spiking insulin better) keeps them off our top-tier list. Otherwise, consuming these whole fruits for fiber, lower calories, and other nutrients may at times be more beneficial for weight gain.

3. Vitamin E

This fat-soluble vitamin is also an antioxidant. It's essential for health and is beneficial for recovery and performance. In fact, a study conducted shows that Vitamin E helps protect cells against damage.

Vitamin E is a very powerful antioxidant that works to protect the integrity of cells in the body. Exercise and intense training produce free radicals in the body, which are toxic by-products of cellular respiration.

As these free radicals accumulate, the body becomes more toxic, causing impaired performance, muscle growth, recovery, and immune health. Vitamin E works to attack these free radicals and flush them out of the body. The result is less oxidative stress and a decrease in muscle damage.

Vitamin E may also help prevent the oxidation of LDL or "bad" cholesterol, which contributes to plaque buildup in the arteries. It boosts the immune system and may reduce the risk of cataracts. Vitamin E also plays a role in healthy skin and hair. Vitamin E can be supplemented without risk of toxicity, unlike other fat-soluble vitamins.

Vitamin E Dosage

Take 400-800 international units (IU) of vitamin E with food each day.

Best Food Sources of Vitamin E

Wheat germ, whole grain products, seed (especially sunflower seeds), nuts (especially hazelnuts and almonds), spinach, and other dark green, leafy vegetables.

4. Magnesium

Athletes and bodybuilders who perform long, intense bouts of exercise lose fluids through sweat, but they also lose key minerals such as magnesium. Magnesium plays a role in maintaining healthy bones and a healthy heart.

The average person needs about 400 milligrams of magnesium a day, but most people consume just over 300 milligrams.

Deficiency can lead to a host of problems, including an increased risk for diabetes and colon cancer. Bodybuilders who are concerned about optimizing their results and performance in the gym, and those who perform intense bouts of exercise should consider supplementing magnesium or focus on obtaining foods rich in this essential mineral.

Magnesium Dosage

Take two 400 milligram dosages per day with food. Keep in mind that calcium and magnesium compete for absorption, so it is best to take magnesium at times when you are consuming low amounts of calcium.

Best Food Sources of Magnesium

Whole-grain bread, cereals, pasta and beans, nuts (almonds and cashews), spinach, soy milk, avocado, and cooked brown rice. Fresh fruits and vegetables also provide a modest amount of magnesium.

The greatest amount of magnesium is found in unprocessed foods.

5. Water

Water itself is not a "nutrient" per se, but it's crucial to health and often contains significant amounts of other macronutrients, particularly essential minerals.

Drinking lots of beverages, especially water, is key to maintaining the fluid balance within your body.

While bodybuilders may like to believe that the bulk of their mass is muscle tissue. In reality, the human body is made of 50%-75% water. According to a Dietetic Association's Complete Food and Nutrition Guide, the average adult loses about 10 cups of water daily. Therefore, replenishing your body's water supply each day is crucial for proper function.

if you are a hard training bodybuilder, it is recommended to consume even more water. While water is of crucial importance to every bodybuilder, we have placed it somewhat lower on this list because the emphasis here is on the macronutrients aspect of water consumption.

The importance of water and other fluids to performance and results is very critical.

Water Dosage

A hard-training bodybuilder should consume at least four liters of water every day and more when performing intense workouts, especially cardio, and at other times when you are sweating a lot. This dosage can be different for bodybuilders cutting weight as water consumption can add more weight.

Best Sources for Water

Tap Water, purified bottled water, tea, coffee, milk, and fruits and vegetables, particularly lettuce, watermelon, broccoli, grapefruit, and apples.

6. Beta-Carotene

Beta-carotene is a plant-based form of vitamin A. It's a preferred form for taking in vitamin A in supplement or food form because it doesn't contain the risk of toxicity that vitamin A supplementation poses in large, frequent doses.

Colorful fruits and vegetables are excellent sources of beta-carotene and pose no risk for overdosing. Beta-carotene is a fat-soluble vitamin, meaning that your body can hold onto it for much longer periods of time than it can with water-soluble vitamins such as vitamin C (because fat-soluble vitamins can be stored in fat tissue).

Beta-carotene is also an antioxidant, so it provides specific recovery benefits for those on hard-training weight programs that produce harmful free radicals.

Beta-Carotene Dosage

Take in up to 4,000 IU of retinol or 5,000 IU of beta-carotene. After supplementing for approximately 4-6 weeks, avoid taking vitamins A for 2-3 weeks to reduce the risk of toxicity.

Best Food Sources of Beta-Carotene

Carrot juice, pumpkin, sweet potato, spinach, carrots, collards, kale, and turnip greens.

7. Electrolytes

Electrolytes are charged particles that perform many functions within the body, one of the most important to regulate the influx and outflow of nutrients and fluids within cells and body tissues. These electrolytes actually function a bit like tiny electrical appliances; when your body runs low on electrolytes it ceases to function as efficiently.

When you are working out, your body produces sweat to cool down the body, your body loses important essential electrolytes such as salt and potassium when sweating.

Supplementing with electrolytes in the form of sports drinks such as Gatorade or Powerade can help prevent your body from getting into an electrolyte deficit. However, keep in mind that many people consume too much sodium (salt) while not getting enough potassium.

You have heard that processed or fast-food diets are extremely high in salts, having too much sodium in your diets can create water retention in your muscles and showing that bloated look. Consume foods that are high in potassium, or consider supplementing with it for best results.

Electrolytes Dosage

Keep your sodium consumption to around 2,000 milligrams or less per day. Dieting bodybuilders can almost completely cut sodium when they are trying to drop water for a bodybuilding contest. You should strive to get about 4,700 milligrams of potassium per day.

Best Food Sources of Electrolytes

Good potassium sources include tomato products, orange juice, beetroot greens, white beans, dates, raisins, baked potatoes, soybeans, and lima beans. Bananas, which are famous for their potassium content, are merely a good source of potassium.

One banana contains about 400 milligrams, compared to 170mL of 100% orange juice, which has over 1,400 milligrams of potassium.

8. Zinc

Zinc is an essential mineral for helping your body maintain a healthy blood supply, but how can it support muscle growth and recovery?. Zinc regulates cell growth, helps heal wounds, and promotes a healthy immune system. It also helps your body use carbohydrates, proteins, and fats for fuel and enhances your sense of taste and smell.

Zinc is also considered beneficial for recovery from stressful exercises such as weight training. However, moderate zinc deficiency is associated with hypogonadism or testosterone deficiency, and since testosterone plays an important role in building and gaining muscles it is important to maintain zinc levels in your body.

The recommended daily intake for zinc is 11 milligrams for men and 8 milligrams for women. These amounts can easily be achieved by consuming a healthful, well-balanced eating plan.

Bodybuilders may need to rely on zinc supplements to get the amount they need based on their increased demands. Be careful with dosage though, zinc is a close balance with copper, and taking in excess may cause your body to lose copper.

Zinc Dosage

Bodybuilders can take up to 30 milligrams as a stand alone or mixed compound supplement such as ZMA.

For best results, take your zinc supplements on an empty stomach about 30 minutes before you go to bed.

Best Food Sources for Zinc

Good sources of zinc include foods of animal origin such as meats and seafood. Eggs, and milk supply zinc in smaller amounts. Whole grain products, wheat germ, black-eyed peas and fermented soybean paste (miso) also contains zinc, but in a form that's less accessible by the body.

Additionally, don't forget that many foods are excellent sources of particular micronutrients. If you are still finding it hard to gain muscles, visit a general practician and get your blood tested to see which vitamins or minerals your body is lacking.

SECTION IV: BUILDING YOUR WEIGHT GAIN MEAL PLAN

BREAKFAST OPTIONS FOR WEIGHT GAIN

Florentine Hash Skillet

Ingredients

• 1 teaspoon extra-virgin olive oil

• 1/2 cup frozen hash browns or precooked shredded potatoes (see Note)

• ½ cup frozen chopped spinach

• 1 large egg

• Pinch of salt

• Pinch of freshly ground pepper

• 2 tablespoons shredded sharp Cheddar cheese

Directions

1. Heat oil in a small nonstick skillet over medium heat. Layer hash browns and spinach into the pan. Crack egg on top and sprinkle with salt, pepper and cheese. Cover, reduce heat to medium-low and cook until the hash browns are starting to brown on the bottom, the egg is set and the cheese is melted, 4 to 7 minutes.

Ricotta & Yogurt Parfait

Ingredients

• ¾ cup nonfat vanilla Greek yogurt

• ¼ cup part-skim ricotta

• ½ teaspoon lemon zest

- ¼ cup raspberries

- 1 tablespoon slivered almonds

- 1 teaspoon chia seeds

Directions

1. Combine yogurt, ricotta and lemon zest in a bowl. Top with raspberries, almonds and chia seeds.

Peanut Butter-Banana Cinnamon Toast

Ingredients

- 1 slice whole-wheat bread, toasted

- 1 tablespoon peanut butter

- 1 small banana, sliced

- Cinnamon, to taste

Directions

1. Spread toast with peanut butter and top with banana slices. Sprinkle with cinnamon to taste.

Spinach & Egg Scramble with Raspberries

Ingredients

• 1 teaspoon canola oil

• 1 ½ cups baby spinach (1 1/2 ounces)

• 2 large eggs, lightly beaten

• Pinch of kosher salt

• Pinch of ground pepper

• 1 slice whole-grain bread, toasted

• ½ cup fresh raspberries

Directions

1. Heat oil in a small nonstick skillet over medium-high heat. Add spinach and cook until wilted, stirring often, 1 to 2 minutes. Transfer the spinach to a plate. Wipe the pan clean, place over medium heat and add eggs. Cook, stirring once or twice to ensure even cooking, until just set, 1 to 2 minutes. Stir in the spinach, salt and pepper. Serve the scramble with toast and raspberries.

Fruit & Yogurt Smoothie

Ingredients

• 3/4 cup nonfat plain yogurt

• 1/2 cup 100% pure fruit juice

• 1 1/2 cups (6 1/2 ounces) frozen fruit, such as blueberries, raspberries, pineapple or peaches

Directions

1. Puree yogurt with juice in a blender until smooth. With the motor running, add fruit through the hole in the lid and continue to puree until smooth.

Everything Bagel Avocado Toast

Ingredients

- ¼ medium avocado, mashed

- 1 slice whole-grain bread, toasted

- 2 teaspoons everything bagel seasoning

- Pinch of flaky sea salt (such as Maldon)

Directions

1. Spread avocado on toast. Top with seasoning and salt.

Muesli with Raspberries

Ingredients

- ⅓ cup muesli

- 1 cup raspberries

- ¾ cup low-fat milk

Directions

1. Top muesli with raspberries and serve with milk.

Pineapple Green Smoothie

Ingredients

- ½ cup unsweetened almond milk

- ⅓ cup nonfat plain Greek yogurt

- 1 cup baby spinach

- 1 cup frozen banana slices (about 1 medium banana)

- ½ cup frozen pineapple chunks

- 1 tablespoon chia seeds

- 1-2 teaspoons pure maple syrup or honey (optional)

Directions

1. Add almond milk and yogurt to a blender, then add spinach, banana, pineapple, chia seeds and sweetener (if using); blend until smooth.

Avocado-Egg Toast

Ingredients

- ¼ avocado

- ¼ teaspoon ground pepper

- ⅛ teaspoon garlic powder

- 1 slice whole-wheat bread, toasted

- 1 large egg, fried

- 1 teaspoon Sriracha (Optional)

- 1 tablespoon scallion, sliced (Optional)

Directions

1. Combine avocado, pepper and garlic powder in a small bowl and gently mash.

2. Top toast with the avocado mixture and fried egg. Garnish with Sriracha and scallion, if desired.

Strawberry-Pineapple Smoothie

Ingredients

- 1 cup frozen strawberries

- 1 cup chopped fresh pineapple

- ¾ cup chilled unsweetened almond milk, plus more if needed

- 1 tablespoon almond butter

Directions

1. Combine strawberries, pineapple, almond milk and almond butter in a blender. Process until smooth, adding more almond milk, if needed, for desired consistency. Serve immediately.

Peanut Butter and Banana Breakfast Sandwich

Ingredients

• 2 slices 100% whole wheat with honey bread

• 4 teaspoons reduced-fat creamy peanut butter

• 1 very small banana or 1/2 of a medium banana, sliced

Directions

1. Toast bread. While toast is still warm, spread 2 teaspoons of the peanut butter on each slice. Arrange banana slices on one of the slices of peanut butter toast. Top with the other slice, peanut butter side down, to make a sandwich.

White Bean & Avocado Toast

Ingredients

- 1 slice whole-wheat bread, toasted

- ¼ avocado, mashed

- ½ cup canned white beans, rinsed and drained

- Kosher salt to taste

- Ground pepper to taste

- 1 pinch Crushed red pepper

Directions

1. Top toast with mashed avocado and white beans. Season with a pinch each of salt, pepper and crushed red pepper.

Peanut Butter & Chia Berry Jam English Muffin

Ingredients

- ½ cup unsweetened mixed frozen berries

- 2 teaspoons chia seeds

- 2 teaspoons natural peanut butter

- 1 whole-wheat English muffin, toasted

Directions

1. Microwave berries in a medium microwave-safe bowl for 30 seconds; stir and microwave 30 seconds more. Stir in chia seeds.

Quick-Cooking Oats

Ingredients

- 1 cup water or low-fat milk

- Pinch of salt

• ½ cup quick-cooking oats (see Tip)

• 1 ounce low-fat milk for serving

• 1 to 2 teaspoons honey, cane sugar or brown sugar for serving

• Pinch of cinnamon

Directions

1. Stovetop: Combine water (or milk) and salt in a small saucepan. Bring to a boil. Stir in oats and reduce heat to medium; cook for 1 minute. Remove from heat, cover and let stand for 2 to 3 minutes.

2. Microwave: Combine water (or milk), salt and oats in a 2-cup microwave-safe bowl. Microwave on High for 1 1/2 to 2 minutes. Stir before serving.

3. Serve with your favorite toppings, such as milk, sweetener, cinnamon, dried fruits and nuts.

Mermaid Smoothie Bowl

Ingredients

- 2 frozen bananas, peeled

- 2 kiwis, peeled

- 1 cup fresh pineapple chunks

- 1 cup unsweetened almond milk

- 2 teaspoons blue spirulina powder

- ½ cup fresh blueberries

- ½ small Fuji apple, thinly sliced and cut into 1-inch flower shapes

Directions

1. Combine bananas, kiwis, pineapple, almond milk and spirulina in a blender. Blend on high until smooth, about 2 minutes.

2. Divide the smoothie between 2 bowls. Top with blueberries and apples.

Egg Salad Avocado Toast

Ingredients

- ¼ avocado

- 1 tablespoon celery

- ½ teaspoon lemon juice

- ½ teaspoon hot sauce

- Pinch of salt

- 1 chopped hard-boiled egg

- 1 slice whole-wheat toast

Directions

1. Mash avocado with celery, lemon juice, hot sauce and salt in a small bowl. Mix in hard-boiled egg. Spread on toast.

Strawberry & Yogurt Parfait

Ingredients

- 1 cup sliced fresh strawberries

- 1 teaspoon sugar

- ½ cup nonfat plain Greek yogurt

- ¼ cup granola

Directions

1. Combine strawberries and sugar in a small bowl and let stand until the berries start to release juice, about 5 minutes.

2. To assemble parfait, layer yogurt and the strawberries with their juice in a 2-cup container. Top with granola.

Raspberry-Kefir Power Smoothie

Ingredients

• ½ frozen banana

• ½ cup raspberries, fresh or frozen

• ⅓ cup low-fat plain kefir

• 2 teaspoons natural peanut butter

• ½ teaspoon flaxmeal

• 1 tablespoon 1-2 tablespoons water

Directions

1. Combine banana, raspberries, kefir, peanut butter and flaxmeal in a blender. Process until smooth, adding water a tablespoon at a time, if necessary.

LUNCH RECIPES TO SUPPORT MUSCLE MASS

Roasted carrot & whipped feta tart

Ingredients

• large bunch of carrots with tops (about 800g)

• 2 tsp olive oil

• 1 tsp za'atar

• 2 tsp honey

• 125-150ml extra virgin olive oil

• 2 garlic cloves, roughly chopped

• 50g walnuts, roughly chopped

• 40g grated parmesan or vegetarian hard cheese

• 25g parsley, roughly chopped, plus whole leaves to serve

• 200g feta drained and crumbled (vegetarian, if needed)

• 150g Greek yogurt

• 1 lemon, zested

• 500g block puff pastry

• 1 egg, beaten

Directions

• STEP 1

Heat the oven to 200C/180C fan/gas 6. Trim off the carrot tops, discarding any tough stems, then set aside.

Halve the carrots lengthways, tip into a roasting tin and toss with the olive oil and some seasoning. Roast for 25-30 mins until tender and golden, stirring once or twice to ensure they don't stick. Stir in the za'atar and honey, and set aside.

• STEP 2

Meanwhile, tip the reserved carrot tops and extra virgin olive oil into a food processor. Season and blitz, scraping down the sides occasionally until finely chopped. Add the garlic, walnuts, parmesan and parsley, and pulse until combined. Pour in another splash of olive oil, if needed. Transfer to a bowl and season to taste. Clean out the food processor, then tip in the feta, yogurt, most of the lemon zest and some seasoning. Blitz until smooth and creamy.

• STEP 3

Put a large baking tray in the oven to heat up. Roll the pastry out on a sheet of baking parchment into a roughly 40 x 30cm rectangle. Gently score a 2cm border around the edge using a sharp knife. Brush the beaten egg all over the pastry and sprinkle a large pinch of sea salt around the border. Carefully slide the pastry onto the hot baking tray using the parchment to help you, and bake for 15-20 mins until golden and puffed up. Remove from the oven and gently press the middle down using the back of a metal spoon. Cool for 5-10 mins, then spread the whipped feta over the middle and arrange the roasted carrots on top. Drizzle over the pesto, scatter over the parsley and the remaining lemon zest, and cut into slices to serve.

Prawn, pancetta & watercress risotto

Ingredients

- 1 tbsp olive oil, plus 1 tsp

- 3 slices pancetta

- 1 large onion, finely chopped

• 200g risotto rice

• 2 garlic cloves, crushed

• 1l hot vegetable stock

• 200g watercress, stalks chopped

• 25g parmesan, finely grated, plus extra to serve

• ½ lemon, zested and juiced

• 180g raw king prawns, peeled and deveined

Directions

• STEP 1

Heat 1 tbsp oil in a wide pan and fry the pancetta for 2 mins on each side. Drain on kitchen paper, then crumble. Fry the onion in the same pan for 5 mins until soft.

• STEP 2

Stir in the rice and garlic for 2 mins to coat in the oil. Add half the stock, bring to the boil and simmer for 5 mins until absorbed. Add the remaining stock, a ladleful at a time, constantly stirring until the rice is tender, about 20 mins.

• STEP 3

Stir in most of the watercress and the parmesan. Season well. Add the lemon zest and a squeeze of juice.

• STEP 4

Spoon half the risotto onto a plate (use for lunch the next day, see tip below). Add the prawns to the pan and cook for 2 mins until pink. Toss the rest of the watercress with 1 tsp oil and lemon juice. Serve over the risotto with some pancetta and parmesan.

Healthy egg & chips

Ingredients

- 500g potatoes, diced

- 2 shallots, sliced

- 1 tbsp olive oil

- 2 tsp dried crushed oregano or 1 tsp fresh leaves

- 200g small mushroom

- 4 eggs

Directions

- STEP 1

Heat oven to 200C/fan 180C/gas 6. Tip the potatoes and shallots into a large, non-stick roasting tin, drizzle with the oil, sprinkle over the oregano, then mix everything together well. Bake for 40-45 mins (or until starting to go brown), add the mushrooms, then cook for a further 10 mins until the potatoes are browned and tender.

• STEP 2

Make four gaps in the vegetables and crack an egg into each space. Return to the oven for 3-4 mins or until the eggs are cooked to your liking.

Minty roast veg & hummus salad

Ingredients

• 4 parsnips, peeled and cut into wedges

• 4 carrots, cut into wedges

• 2 tsp cumin seeds

- 400g can chickpeas, drained

- 2 tbsp vegetable oil

- 500g pack cooked beetroot (not in vinegar), drained and cut into wedges

- 2 tbsp clear honey

- 200g pot hummus

- 2 tbsp white wine vinegar

- small bunch mint, leaves picked

- 200g block Greek-style salad cheese or feta

Directions

- STEP 1

Heat oven to 200C/180C fan/gas 6. Toss the parsnips, carrots, cumin seeds and chickpeas with the oil and some seasoning in a large roasting tin. Cook for 30 mins, tossing halfway through cooking.

• STEP 2

Add the beetroot to the tin and drizzle over the honey, then return to the oven for 10 mins. Spread the hummus thinly over a large platter, or divide between 4 dinner plates. When the veg is ready, drizzle with the vinegar and toss together in the tin. Tip the roasted vegetables on top of the hummus, scatter over the mint and cheese, drizzle with any juices from the tin and serve.

Easy chocolate brownie cake

Ingredients

• 175g unsalted butter, plus extra for greasing

• 225g dark chocolate, broken into pieces

• 200g caster sugar

• 3 medium eggs, separated

• 65g plain flour

• 50g chopped pecan nuts

Directions

• STEP 1

Heat oven to 180C/fan 160C/gas 4. Butter a 20-25cm cake tin and line with greaseproof paper.

• STEP 2

Place 175g/6oz of the chocolate, plus the butter and sugar in a heavy-based pan and heat gently until melted, stirring occasionally. Leave to cool.

• STEP 3

Whisk the egg yolks into the chocolate mixture, then add the flour, nuts and the remaining chocolate.

• STEP 4

Whisk the egg whites until they form soft peaks, then gently, but thoroughly, fold into the chocolate mixture.

• STEP 5

Pour into the prepared tin and bake in the centre of the oven for about 35-40 mins until crusty on top. Leave to cool, then run a knife around the sides and remove from the tin. Dust with icing sugar and serve warm with custard or ice cream or cold with cream.

Saag paneer

Ingredients

- 2 tbsp ghee, or cooking oil

- 1 tsp turmeric

- 1 tsp chilli powder or Kashmiri chilli powder

- 450g paneer, cut into 3cm cubes

- 500g spinach, mature fresh or frozen

- 1 large onion, finely chopped

- 3 garlic cloves

- thumb-sized piece of ginger

- 1 green chilli, roughly chopped, (include seeds for extra spice)

- 1 tsp garam masala

- ½ lemon, juiced, to serve

Directions

• STEP 1

Melt the ghee, whisk in with the turmeric and chilli powder, then add the cubed paneer and toss well. Set aside. If using frozen spinach, microwave for 3-5 mins, then place in a sieve and squeeze out most of the water. If using fresh spinach, place in a colander, pour over boiling water, drain and cool, then put in a tea towel and squeeze out most of the water. Roughly chop.

• STEP 2

Blitz the onion with the garlic, ginger and green chilli. Cook the paneer in a large non-stick frying pan over medium heat for around 8 mins, tossing the pan so they become golden all over. Remove and set aside on a plate, leaving spices behind in the pan. Tip the onion mix into the pan, add a pinch of salt and turn the heat down. Fry until caramel coloured, around 10 mins, adding a splash of water if it looks a little dry. Add the garam masala, stir to coat the onion mix, fry for 2 mins.

• STEP 3

Add the spinach and cook for a further 2-3 mins, adding 100ml water to release all the flavours from the bottom of the pan. Season to taste. Add the paneer and cook for 2-3 mins to heat through. Spoon into bowls and squeeze over a little lemon juice, to serve.

Pad Thai

Ingredients

• 250g pack medium rice noodle

• 2 tsp tamarind paste

• 3 tbsp fish sauce

• 2 tsp sugar

* 1 garlic clove

* 3 spring onions

* 2 tbsp vegetable oil

* 1 egg

* 200g pack large cooked prawn

* 75g beansprout

* handful salted peanut, chopped to serve

* lime wedges, to serve

Directions

* STEP 1

Tip the noodles into a large bowl and pour over a kettle of boiling water until they are covered. Leave to stand for 5-10 mins until the noodles are soft, then drain well. (You can do this part ahead of time – then just run the noodles under cold water until cool, and toss through a little oil to stop them from sticking.) Next, mix together the tamarind paste, fish sauce and sugar in a small bowl.

• STEP 2

Peel and finely chop the garlic. Trim the ends off the spring onions and cut into thin slices about 1cm long. Heat a wok or large frying pan over a high heat. When it's really hot (a drop of water should sizzle straight away), pour in the oil and swirl around. Tip in garlic and spring onions. To stir-fry, take a spatula or tongs and toss the veg around the wok so they're moving all the time. Cook for 30 secs, just until they begin to soften.

• STEP 3

Push the vegetables to the sides of the wok, then crack the egg into the centre. Keep stirring the egg for 30 secs until it begins to set and resembles a broken-up omelette.

• STEP 4

Add the prawns and beansprouts, followed by the noodles, then pour over the fish sauce mixture. Toss everything together and heat through. Spoon out onto plates. Serve with some chopped peanuts sprinkled over and wedges of lime.

Red lentil & coconut soup

Ingredients

• 100g red lentils

• 1 heaped tsp turmeric

• 1 tbsp coarsely grated ginger

* 2 garlic cloves, sliced

* 1l vegetable stock

* 400ml can coconut milk

* 2 leeks, well washed and sliced

* 2 handfuls baby spinach (approx 50g/2oz)

Supercharged topping

* 2 limes, cut into wedge

Directions

* STEP 1

Tip the lentils into a large pan and add the turmeric, ginger and garlic. Pour in the stock, then cover the pan and simmer for 15 mins until the lentils have softened.

- STEP 2

Pour in the coconut milk, stir in the leeks, cover and cook for 10 mins more.

- STEP 3

Add the spinach and cook just to wilt it, then spoon into bowls and squeeze over the lime juice.

Roast turkey breast

Ingredients

- 1 large single turkey breast or 1 double breast tied into a joint (about 2kg in total)

- 2 large onions, thickly sliced

- 2 large carrots, cut into 4 horizontal slices

- 20g butter, at room temperature

Directions

• STEP 1

Take the turkey breast out of the fridge and allow it to come to room temperature for an hour.

• STEP 2

Heat the oven to 190C/170C fan/gas 5. Put a rack inside an oven tray with the onions and carrots underneath, or arrange the veg inside an ovenproof frying pan.

• STEP 3

Weigh the turkey breast and calculate 40 mins per kilo, plus an additional 20 mins.

• STEP 4

Rub the butter over the skin and season well. Put the turkey breast on the rack or rest it on top of the veg in the pan.

• STEP 5

Pour in enough water to cover the veg and cover the whole tin or pan with a tent of foil.

• STEP 6

Roast for the allotted time, taking the foil off 20 mins before the end to brown the skin. Test with the point of a knife and see if the point feels hot as soon as you pull it out (be careful) and the juices run clear. If you have a thermometer then it should read 65-70C. If the joint appears to be underdone, then put back in the oven for another 10 mins.

• STEP 7

Leave the turkey to rest for 20 mins somewhere warm, it will keep cooking so the final internal temperature will rise to 70C, or just above that. Don't skip this step otherwise the juices will run out as you carve.

• STEP 8

Use the strained veg and liquid in the bottom of the tin and the juices from carving to add to this gravy, if you like, and serve with the turkey and veg.

Sticky slow-roast belly of pork

Ingredients

• 1.3kg piece pork belly, boned, rind left on and scored (ask your butcher to do this)

• 2 tsp sunflower oil

• 1 tsp white peppercorns, crushed

• 3 large onions, sliced

• 2-3 tbsp clear honey

• 2 tsp ground cumin

• 1 red chilli, deseeded and chopped

Directions

• STEP 1

Heat oven to 180C/fan 160C/gas 4. Lay the pork, skin-side up, on a rack in a roasting tin. Trickle with a little oil, then lightly press on the crushed peppercorns and a sprinkling of coarse sea salt. Place in the oven, then cook for 1 hr. Remove from the oven and baste with the juices. Continue to cook for a further 1½ hrs, basting every 20 mins.

• STEP 2

Put the sliced onions in the roasting tin under the pork. Mix the honey together with the cumin and chilli, brush it over the pork, then increase the oven to 200C/fan 180C/ gas 6. Cook for a further 30-40 mins, basting occasionally, until caramelised with a rich, golden glaze over the pork. Once cooked and tender (this can be easily tested by piercing the flesh with a knife), remove pork from the oven, then leave to rest for 10-15 mins.

• STEP 3

While the pork is resting, heat the tin on the stove with the onions, adding 2 tbsp water. This will lift any residue from the pan, creating a moist cooking liquor. Season the onions with salt and pepper, then divide between 6 plates. Carve pork into 6 portions, then serve on top of the onions. Pour any remaining liquor over and serve with the Pumpkin mash

RECIPE TIPS

PUMPKIN MASH

Peel 1 kg pumpkin and cut into chunks. Season and roast with the

pork for the last 30 mins until soft and fluffy. Meanwhile, peel 1kg potatoes and cut into chunks. Boil in salted water

for 10 mins until soft. Drain and mash with 2 tbsp

milk and 50g butter, seasoning to taste. Mash the

pumpkin into the potato until smooth.

Roasted veg & couscous salad

Ingredients

• 1 red and 1 yellow pepper, halved and deseeded

• ½ butternut squash

- 2 courgettes, thickly sliced

- 4 garlic cloves, leave skin on

- 3 tbsp extra-virgin olive oil

- 1 red onion, thickly sliced

- 1 tsp cumin seeds

- 1 tbsp harissa paste

- 50g whole blanched almonds

- 250g couscous

- 300ml hot vegetable stock

- zest and juice 1 lemon

- 20g pack mint, roughly chopped

Directions

• STEP 1

Heat oven to 200C/180C fan/gas 6. Cut peppers and squash into bite-size pieces (leave skin on the squash). Tip all the veg into a baking tray, add garlic, 2 tbsp oil and seasoning, then mix and roast for 20 mins. Add onion, cumin, harissa and almonds. Roast for another 20 mins, then cool.

• STEP 2

Put couscous into a large bowl, pour over the stock, cover, then set aside for 10 mins. Fluff up with a fork.

• STEP 3

In a bowl, mix zest, juice and remaining oil. Squeeze garlic pulp from skins into the bowl, mash well and fold in the mint. Pour over the veg, then toss with the couscous.

Mango chutney baked feta with lentils

Ingredients

• 200g pack feta

• 1 tbsp mango chutney

• 150ml natural yogurt

• small handful mint, finely chopped

• small handful dill, finely chopped, plus extra fronds to serve

• 1 tbsp olive oil

• 250g pack microwave puy lentils

• ½ medium cucumber, halved, deseeded and cut into half-moons

• 120g cherry tomatoes, halved

Directions

• STEP 1

Heat oven to 220C/200C fan/ gas 7. Put the feta in an ovenproof dish and spread over the mango chutney. Bake for about 20 mins until sticky.

• STEP 2

Mix the yogurt, half the mint, half the dill, the olive oil and 1 tbsp water to make a dressing. Season to taste.

• STEP 3

Cook the lentils in the microwave according to pack instructions. Toss the lentils with the cucumber and tomatoes. Divide between two plates and top with the feta, a drizzle of the yogurt dressing and any remaining herbs.

Sriracha-glazed chicken burger & pickled cabbage

Ingredients

• 4 large, boneless and skinless chicken thighs

• 2 garlic cloves, finely grated or crushed

• 1 tsp smoked paprika

• pinch chilli flakes

• thumb-sized piece ginger, finely grated

• 4 brioche burger buns, halved, to serve

For the pickled cabbage

• 150ml cider vinegar

• 75g golden caster sugar

- ½ tsp coriander seeds

- 1 tsp ground turmeric

- ½ Chinese cabbage or pointed cabbage, shredded

For the relish

- ¼ cucumber, coarsely grated

- 3 tbsp mayonnaise

- 1 lime, zested and juiced

For the glaze

- 3 tbsp American mustard

- 2 tbsp sriracha

Directions

- STEP 1

Flatten the chicken thighs out by lightly bashing them between two pieces of baking parchment with a rolling pin, then put in a sealable container with the garlic, paprika, chilli, ginger and a pinch of salt. Massage the mix into the meat, then chill until ready to cook for at least 1 hr or up to 24 hrs.

• STEP 2

To pickle the cabbage, put the vinegar, sugar, coriander seeds and turmeric in a pan and bring to the boil to dissolve the sugar. Take off the heat and stir in the shredded cabbage, ensuring it's completely immersed in the liquid. Cover and leave to cool.

• STEP 3

For the relish, sprinkle the cucumber with a little salt and leave for 10 mins. Squeeze out the liquid, then stir the cucumber through the mayo and lime juice and set aside. For the glaze, mix the mustard and sriracha together in a separate bowl.

• STEP 4

Heat a barbecue to medium or the grill to its highest setting. Barbecue or grill the chicken for 5 mins on one side, then flip and continue to cook, brushing with the glaze a few times until sticky, glossy and cooked through. Toast the buns, spoon some cabbage onto the base, place the chicken on top, then dollop a generous amount of the cooling cucumber relish over the chicken before closing the buns and serving.

Spring one-pot roast chicken

Ingredients

• 1 ½kg whole chicken

• 250g mascarpone

• ½ small lemon, zested and juiced

• small bunch of tarragon, finely chopped

• 3 tbsp olive oil

• 800g new potatoes, halved if large

• 1 garlic bulb, halved

• 200g radishes, halved if large

• ½ bunch of spring onions, trimmed

• 150ml chicken stock

• 200g frozen peas, defrosted

• 100g spring greens, shredded

Directions

• STEP 1

Heat the oven to 200C/180C fan/gas 6. Remove any string from the chicken and sit in a large roasting tin or a baking dish, with plenty of space around it.

• STEP 2

Mash 2 tbsp of the mascarpone with the lemon zest, 1 tbsp of the tarragon and some seasoning. Slip your hand beneath the chicken skin to pull it away from the meat, then spread the mixture beneath the skin in a thin layer. Spoon another 3 tbsp mascarpone into the cavity of the chicken, to melt in with the roasting juices and enrich the sauce later on. Rub 2 tbsp olive oil into the skin, season well with sea salt, then loosely tie the legs together with butcher's string. Roast for 20 mins.

• STEP 3

Arrange the potatoes and the garlic around the chicken, drizzle over another 1 tbsp oil and cook for another 30 mins.

• STEP 4

Toss the radishes and whole spring onions into the dish, in and around the potatoes, coating everything in the fat, then roast for another 25 mins. The potatoes and radishes will be golden and tender, and the chicken should be cooked through. Remove the chicken from the tin, cover loosely with foil and leave to rest.

• STEP 5

Pour off or spoon away the excess oil from the tin. Stir the remaining mascarpone (about 150g) with the stock in a jug until lump-free, then pour into the tin and bubble on the hob for few minutes, stirring to coat the potatoes and veg. Squeeze over some lemon juice and season.

• STEP 6

Stir in the peas, spring greens and most of the remaining tarragon, and bubble for a few more minutes until bright green. Sit the chicken back in the middle of the tin to serve and scatter over the reserved tarragon.

Sticky treacle-glazed ham

Ingredients

• 3.5-4kg/7lb 10oz-9lb boned rolled piece unsmoked ham

• 2 oranges, 1 cut into wedges and finely grated zest and juice of the other

• 1 cinnamon stick

• 2 tbsp English mustard

• 85g black treacle

• handful cloves

• big bunch bay leaves and orange segments, to serve (optional)

Directions

• STEP 1

If you need to soak the ham, do so the night before. Heat oven to 180C/fan 160C/gas 4. Place the ham, skin-side up, in a deep roasting tin, then add enough water to cover the base of the tin. Scatter the orange wedges and cinnamon stick around. Cover the pan with a tight tent of foil, then cook the ham for about 2½ hrs. (If using a different weight of ham, you want 20 mins per 450g.)

• STEP 2

While the ham is cooking, mix the mustard, treacle and orange zest together with enough orange juice to make a mixture loose enough to paint over the ham.

• STEP 3

When the ham has had its time, remove the roasting tin from the oven and turn up the heat to 220C/ fan 200C/gas 7. Remove the foil, leave the ham until cool enough to handle, then pour away any liquid in the tin. Using a sharp knife, carefully cut away the skin to leave an even layer of fat. Use the tip of the knife to score the ham fat diagonally at 3cm intervals – first in one direction, then the other, to produce a diamond pattern. Liberally paint the glaze over the fat, then stud with the cloves at the points of the diamond shapes.

• STEP 4

Roast the ham for 30 mins until glazed and just beginning to char around the edges. Leave to cool and serve warm or cold, decorated with the bay and orange wedges, if you like, along with my delicious green bean salad and your favourite chutney.

Swedish meatball burgers

Ingredients

- 500g lean beef or pork mince

- 1 onion, coarsely grated

- 1 egg, beaten

- 25g dried breadcrumbs

- grated nutmeg

- ¼ tsp garlic powder

- burger buns, sliced cheese, lettuce, sliced tomato and lingonberry sauce (optional), to serve

Directions

- STEP 1

Tip the mince, onion, egg, breadcrumbs, nutmeg and garlic powder into a large bowl and generously season with black pepper. Mix everything together using your hands, then shape the mixture into six patties. Transfer to a plate, cover and chill for 1 hr or up to a day.

• STEP 2

Heat a barbecue to medium or until a thin layer of coals has turned grey. Cook the burgers for 10 mins, turning occasionally, until lightly charred and cooked through. Top with sliced cheese during the final 2 mins of cooking time, if you like.

• STEP 3

Serve the burgers in the buns topped with the lettuce, tomato and lingonberry sauce, if you like.

Sweet potato, spinach & feta tortilla

Ingredients

• 3 sweet potatoes

• 2 tbsp olive oil

• 100g baby spinach

• 6 large eggs

• 100g feta, crumbled

Directions

• STEP 1

Pierce the potatoes a few times on each side. Microwave on high for 5-8 mins until soft, then set aside to cool a little.

• STEP 2

Heat the oil in a 20cm ovenproof frying pan and wilt the spinach for a minute or two (you might have to do this in batches). Cut each potato in half lengthways and use a spoon to scoop out the flesh, keeping it in big chunks. Whisk the eggs.

• STEP 3

Add the sweet potato to the pan and stir to combine with the spinach – don't break it up too much. Pour in the egg and swirl around so it fills any gaps in the pan. Scatter over the feta and cook for 4-5 mins over a low heat until the bottom and sides are set.

• STEP 4

Place under the grill for 1-2 mins to cook the top – poke a knife into the centre to ensure it's cooked through. Cool before slicing into wedges. Will keep chilled for up to a day.

Yaki udon (stir-fried udon noodles)

Ingredients

- 250g dried udon noodles (400g frozen or fresh)

- 2 tbsp sesame oil

- 1 onion, thickly sliced

- ¼ head white cabbage, roughly sliced

- 10 shiitake mushrooms

- 4 spring onions, finely sliced

For the sauce

- 4 tbsp mirin

- 2 tbsp soy sauce

- 1 tbsp caster sugar

- 1 tbsp Worcestershire sauce (or vegetarian alternative)

Directions

• STEP 1

Boil some water in a large saucepan. Add 250ml cold water and the udon noodles. (As they are so thick, adding cold water helps them to cook a little bit slower so the middle cooks through). If using frozen or fresh noodles, cook for 2 mins or until al dente; dried will take longer, about 5-6 mins. Drain and leave in the colander.

• STEP 2

Heat 1 tbsp of the oil, add the onion and cabbage and sauté for 5 mins until softened. Add the mushrooms and some spring onions, and sauté for 1 more min. Pour in the remaining sesame oil and the noodles. If using cold noodles, let them heat through before adding the **Ingredients** for the sauce – otherwise tip in straight away and keep stir-frying until sticky and piping hot. Sprinkle with the remaining spring onions.

Vegan kale pesto pasta

Ingredients

- 150g kale

- small bunch of basil

- 1 small garlic clove

- 3 tbsp pumpkin seeds

- 5 tbsp extra virgin olive oil

- 3 tbsp nutritional yeast

- 1 lemon, zested and juiced

- 350g wholemeal spaghetti

Directions

• STEP 1

Bring a pan of water to the boil. Cook the kale for 30 secs, drain and transfer to a bowl of ice-cold water for 5 mins. Drain again and pat dry with kitchen paper.

• STEP 2

Put the basil, garlic, seeds, oil, nutritional yeast, lemon juice and zest, and drained kale in a food processor. Blitz until smooth, then season. Loosen with a splash of water, if it's too thick.

• STEP 3

Cook the pasta following pack instructions, then toss with the pesto and serve.

Chorizo & chickpea soup

Ingredients

- 400g can chopped tomato

- 110g pack of chorizo sausage (unsliced)

- 140g wedge Savoy cabbage

- sprinkling dried chilli flakes

- 410g can chickpea, drained and rinsed

- 1 chicken or vegetable stock cube

- crusty bread or garlic bread, to serve

Directions

- STEP 1

Put a medium pan on the heat and tip in the tomatoes, followed by a can of water. While the tomatoes are heating, quickly chop the chorizo into chunky pieces (removing any skin) and shred the cabbage.

• STEP 2

Pile the chorizo and cabbage into the pan with the chilli flakes and chickpeas, then crumble in the stock cube. Stir well, cover and leave to bubble over a high heat for 6 mins or until the cabbage is just tender. Ladle into bowls and eat with crusty or garlic bread.

Mushrooms on toast

Ingredients

• 4 large slices sourdough bread

• 1 tbsp olive oil

• 4 slices prosciutto

• knob of butter

• 350g mixed mushrooms

* 1 garlic clove, crushed

* 4 tbsp crème fraîche

* handful parsley leaves, finely chopped

Directions

* STEP 1

Toast the sourdough bread, cut each slice in half, then set aside. Heat a large frying pan with the olive oil. Fry the prosciutto in the pan for about 2 mins on each side until golden and crisp. Break into large pieces and set aside on some kitchen paper.

* STEP 2

Add the butter to the pan followed by the mushrooms. Cook for 2 mins, then add the garlic and crème fraîche. Cook for 3-5 mins more until the mushrooms are soft and lightly coated in the crème fraîche. Stir through a little parsley. Pile up on the toasts and top with the prosciutto and more parsley.

HIGH-CALORIE DINNER OPTIONS

Next level chicken katsu curry

Ingredients

For the katsu

• 2 large chicken breasts

• 400ml milk

• 100g plain flour

• 2 eggs, beaten

• 150g panko breadcrumbs or coarse dried breadcrumbs

• sprinkling shichimi togarashi or chilli power, plus extra to serve

- splash of soy sauce

- sunflower oil, for frying

For the curry sauce

- 50g butter

- 1 large carrot, chopped

- 1 onion, chopped

- 4 garlic cloves, chopped

- large piece of ginger, chopped

- 2 tbsp mild curry powder

- 1 tbsp honey

- 1 tbsp ketchup

- 1 tbsp red or brown miso paste

• 1 tbsp soy sauce

• 1 chicken stock cube

• shredded white cabbage, shredded nori, sesame seeds and cooked rice, to serve

Instructions

• STEP 1

Cut each chicken breast in half lengthways, creating four fillets. Put each fillet between two sheets of baking parchment and beat with a rolling pin to even out the thickness.

• STEP 2

Pour the milk into a bowl and season with a large pinch of salt, then add the chicken fillets. Cover and leave in the fridge for at least 20 mins or for up to 24 hrs (the longer you leave the chicken in the milk, the more succulent it will be).

• STEP 3

When you're ready to coat the chicken, tip the flour, eggs and breadcrumbs into three separate bowls, then season the flour with the togarashi and stir the soy sauce into the eggs. Scoop one chicken fillet out of the milk and coat in the flour mix, then dip into the egg mix and coat in the breadcrumbs. Set on a plate and repeat with the rest of the chicken fillets. Can be prepared up to a day ahead and frozen for up to a month.

• STEP 4

To make the curry sauce, heat the butter in a saucepan and sizzle the carrot and onion for 5 mins, then add the garlic and ginger and cook for a few mins more. Scatter over the curry powder and cook for 1 min, then stir in the honey, ketchup, miso paste and soy sauce to create a sticky paste. Cook for 1 min more, then pour in 700ml boiling water and crumble in the stock cube. Cover and simmer for 20 mins until the carrot is soft. Tip the sauce into a blender and blitz until completely smooth (alternatively, use a hand blender). Season to taste. Can be made up to three days ahead and chilled or frozen for up to three months.

• STEP 5

To cook the katsu, heat a good layer of oil in a large frying pan, then add as many of the chicken fillets as you can fit and fry for 3-4 mins on each side until deep golden and crisp. Transfer to a tray and keep warm in a low oven while you cook the remaining fillets.

• STEP 6

Mix the cabbage and seaweed and sprinkle over some sesame seeds, if using. Top the katsu with the curry sauce and serve with the rice and salad, if you like.

Tuna, caper & chilli spaghetti

Ingredients

- 150g spaghetti or linguine

- 1 tbsp olive oil

- 1 garlic clove, sliced

- 1 red chilli, deseeded and finely chopped, plus extra to serve (optional)

- 1 tbsp drained capers

- small bunch of parsley, finely chopped (stalks included)

- 145g tuna in spring water, drained

- 90g rocket or baby spinach leaves

• ½ lemon, juiced

Instructions

• STEP 1

Cook the spaghetti for 9-11 mins in a large pan of well-salted water until al dente.

• STEP 2

Heat the oil in a wide frying pan over a very low heat, and gently cook the garlic and chilli to infuse the oil. Remove from the heat if the garlic is turning past light golden, as this will make it bitter.

• STEP 3

Drain the pasta, keeping a cupful of the cooking water, and tip the spaghetti into the frying pan. Toss the pasta in the oil over a low heat, adding a little of the pasta water to emulsify into a sauce that coats the pasta, then fold in the capers, parsley, tuna and some seasoning. Don't stir too vigorously – you want to keep larger chunks of tuna. Toss the rocket and lemon juice through the spaghetti, and serve with extra chilli scattered over, if you like.

Tomato & courgette risotto

Ingredients

• 2 tbsp olive oil

• 1 small onion, diced

• 2 garlic cloves, crushed

• ½ tsp coriander seeds, crushed

• 200g risotto rice

• 500ml vegetable stock

• 200g carton passata

• 12 cherry tomatoes, halved

• 2 courgettes, halved and sliced

• 2 tbsp mascarpone

• parmesan (or vegetarian alternative), grated, to serve

Instructions

• STEP 1

Put1 tbsp of oil in a large pan over a medium heat. Add the onion and cook for 5-7 mins until softened. Add the garlic and coriander seeds and cook, stirring, for another 1 min. Stir in the risotto rice, coating it in the onion mixture. Gradually add 300ml of the vegetable stock, stirring until fully absorbed by the rice between each addition. Pour the passata into the risotto, cover and simmer for 10-15 mins. Stir occasionally and add more stock as needed.

• STEP 2

Meanwhile, heat oven to 200C/180C fan/gas 6. Put the cherry tomatoes and courgettes in a roasting tin, keeping them separate, drizzle with 1 tbsp olive oil, season and roast for 10-12 mins until just tender.

• STEP 3

Add the mascarpone and plenty of seasoning to the risotto. Stir until the rice is completely cooked and the risotto is creamy, about 5 mins more. Add the courgettes and stir to combine. Serve the risotto in bowls topped with the roasted tomatoes and some grated Parmesan.

Creamy pesto & kale pasta

Ingredients

- 1 tbsp rapeseed oil

- 2 red onions, thinly sliced

- 300g kale

- 300g wholemeal pasta (penne or mafalda work well)

- 4 tbsp reduced-fat soft cheese

- 4 tbsp fresh or jar pesto, or vegetarian alternative

Instructions

- STEP 1

Heat the oil in a large pan over a medium heat. Fry the onions for 10 mins until softened and beginning to caramelise. Add the kale and 100ml water, then cover and cook for 5 mins more, or until the kale has wilted.

- STEP 2

Cook the pasta following pack instructions. Drain, reserving a little of the cooking water. Toss the pasta with the onion mixture, soft cheese and pesto, adding a splash of the reserved cooking water to loosen, if needed. Season.

Crispy grilled feta with saucy butter beans

Ingredients

• 500ml passata

• 2 x 400g cans butter beans, drained and rinsed

• 2 garlic cloves, crushed

• 1 tsp dried oregano, plus a pinch

• 200g spinach

• 2 roasted red peppers, sliced

* ½ lemon, zested and juiced

* 100g block of feta, cut into chunks

* ½ tsp olive oil

* 4 small pittas

Instructions

* STEP 1

Put a large ovenproof frying pan over a medium-high heat, and tip in the passata, butter beans, garlic, oregano, spinach and peppers. Stir together and cook for 6-8 mins until the sauce is bubbling and the spinach has wilted. Season, then add the lemon juice.

* STEP 2

Heat the grill to high. Scatter the feta over the sauce, so it's still exposed, drizzle with the olive oil and sprinkle over the lemon zest plus a pinch of oregano, then grind over some black pepper. Grill for 5-8 mins until the feta is golden and crisp at the edges.

• STEP 3

Meanwhile, toast the pittas under the grill or in the toaster, then serve with the beans and feta.

Carbonara with chicken

Ingredients

• 1 pack spaghetti

• 1 tbsp olive oil

• 1 garlic clove, halved

• 77g pack pancetta

• 1 chicken breast, cut into strips

• 2 eggs

• 100g Grana Padano, finely grated, plus extra to serve (wrap the rest tightly and it will keep for several weeks)

• 1 tbsp butter

Instructions

• STEP 1

Cook the spaghetti following pack instructions. Meanwhile, heat the oil in a frying pan and fry the garlic and pancetta until crisp, then add the chicken strips and fry briefly until they're just cooked through. Fish out the garlic clove and discard it. Beat the eggs with the grana padano and some black pepper.

• STEP 2

Add a couple of tablespoons of pasta water to the pancetta pan along with the butter, then drain the pasta and add it to the pan. Pour in the egg mixture, take the pan off the heat and toss together so the egg cooks in the heat of the pasta. Divide between four warm bowls and top with more cheese, if you like.

Red onion & chilli bhajis with mint & garlic raita

Ingredients

• 2 red onions

• 100g chickpea flour (gram flour)

• ½ tsp baking powder

• 2 tsp curry paste or powder

• 1 red or green chilli, deseeded and finely chopped

• vegetable oil, for frying

For the raita

• 150g tub natural yogurt

• 2 tbsp chopped mint

• 1 small garlic clove, crushed

Instructions

• STEP 1

Finely chop one onion and thinly slice the other. Sift the flour and baking powder into a bowl. Add the curry paste or powder, chopped chilli and a good sprinkling of salt. Add about 150ml of cold water to make a thick batter. Stir in the chopped and sliced onions until they are well coated.

• STEP 2

Mix together the raita Ingredients with a little salt and pepper, then spoon into a small bowl. Heat about 5cm of oil in a wok or deep pan. Add a tiny speck of batter, if it rises to the surface surrounded by bubbles and starts to brown, then the oil is hot enough.

• STEP 3

Add heaped tbsps of onion mix to the pan, a few at a time, and cook for a few mins, turning once, until they are evenly browned and crisp, about 3-4 mins. Drain on kitchen paper, sprinkle with a little salt and keep warm while you cook the remaining bhajis. Serve with the raita.

Slow cooker leg of lamb

Ingredients

• 2 tbsp olive oil

• 1.3kg boneless leg of lamb, tied

- 30g unsalted butter

- 2 tbsp plain flour

- 300ml lamb stock

- 200ml red wine

- 2 red onions, cut into wedges

- 2 garlic cloves, sliced

- 5 sprigs of thyme

- 5 sprigs of rosemary

- mashed potatoes and steamed veg, to serve

Instructions

- STEP 1

Heat the oil in a large non-stick frying pan. Add the lamb and brown on each side for 4-5 mins. Set the slow cooker to low. Melt the butter in a saucepan until foaming, then stir through the flour. Whisk in the stock gradually until incorporated, add the wine and bring to the boil. Set aside.

• STEP 2

Put the onion, garlic, thyme and rosemary into your slow cooker and sit the lamb on top. Pour over the lamb gravy. Put the lid on and cook for 8 hrs or until soft and tender.

• STEP 3

Remove the lamb and set, covered, on a plate. Strain the liquid into a pan and simmer until slightly thickened. Serve the lamb thickly sliced or shredded (it'll be quite soft) with mashed potatoes, green veg and the gravy.

Smoky hake, beans & greens

Ingredients

• mild olive oil

• ½ x 200g pack raw cooking chorizo (we used Unearthed Alfresco Smoked)

• 1 onion, finely chopped

• 260g bag spinach

• 2 x 140g skinless hake fillets

• ½ tsp sweet smoked paprika

• 1 red chilli, deseeded and shredded

• 400g can cannellini beans, drained

• juice ½ lemon

• 1 tbsp extra virgin olive oil

To serve

• Quick garlic mayonnaise (optional)

Instructions

• STEP 1

Boil a full kettle of water and heat the grill to high. Heat 1 tsp oil in a large frying pan. Squeeze the meat from the chorizo directly into the pan. Add the onion and fry for 5 mins, crushing the meat with a spatula until broken up, golden and surrounded by its juices. The onion will also be soft and golden.

• STEP 2

Meanwhile, put the spinach in a colander, slowly pour over the boiled water to wilt it, then run under the cold tap. Squeeze out the excess water using your hands, then set aside. Line a baking tray with foil, rub with a little oil and place the fish on top. Season, sprinkle over the smoked paprika and drizzle with a little more oil.

• STEP 3

Tip the chilli into the pan with the sausages, fry for 1 min more, then add the beans, spinach, lemon juice and extra virgin olive oil. Let it warm through gently, then season to taste.

• STEP 4

Grill the fish for 5 mins or until flaky but not dry – you won't need to turn it. Spoon the bean mixture onto plates, then carefully top with the fish and any juices from the tray. Serve with a dollop of Quick garlic mayonnaise (see recipe, right), if you like.

Tandoori spiced sea bream

Ingredients

- drizzle olive oil, for frying

- 2 sea bream fillets

For the tandoori butter

- 1 tsp garlic paste (blend lots of peeled garlic with a little vegetable oil, then freeze in ice cube trays)

- 1 tsp ginger paste (made as above)

- 2 green chillies

- ¼ tsp red chilli powder

- ½ tsp turmeric

- ½ tsp garam masala

- juice ½ lime

- 100g unsalted butter

Instructions

• STEP 1

Mix the tandoori butter Ingredients, plus some seasoning, in a small food processor or with a hand-held blender until smooth. Scrape onto cling film, then use the cling film to help you roll it into a cylinder. Twist the ends to seal in the butter and chill until firm. The butter will last in the fridge for a week, or in the freezer for up to 3 months.

• STEP 2

Heat a heavy-based frying pan with a drizzle of oil until really hot. Season the fish, then place in the pan, skin-side down, and cook for 4-5 mins until crisp and almost cooked through. Carefully turn over, add a good tbsp of tandoori butter to the pan and spoon it over the fish as it melts. Serve straight away with the Crushed saffron potatoes and Green beans with coconut (recipes below), with any pan juices poured over.

RECIPE TIPS

STRAWBERRY SHORTBREAD CARDAMOM POTS

Whip a small pot double cream with just enough sugar to sweeten. Crush 3-4 cardamom pods to remove the seeds, then finely crush the seeds before stirring into the cream with lots of sliced strawberries and 3-4 crumbled shortbread fingers. Spoon into pretty pots and eat with extra shortbread.

CRUSHED SAFFRON POTATOES

Cook 300g new potatoes in boiling, salted water until tender. Meanwhile, soften a pinch saffron in a drop of warm water. Drain the cooked potatoes and return to the pan over a low heat. Add 25g butter, the saffron and plenty of seasoning. Roughly crush together with a whisk or fork, then serve with the fish.

GREEN BEANS WITH COCONUT

Blanch 140g trimmed green beans in boiling, salted water for 2-3 mins until just tender. Drain and rinse under cold water to cool. Fry 1 tsp black or brown mustard seeds and 2 tbsp unsweetened desiccated coconut in 2 tsp sunflower oil for 1-2 mins until golden and fragrant. Stir in the beans until warmed through, then serve with the fish and potatoes.

Easy roasted cauliflower

Ingredients

• 2 heads cauliflower, cut into even bite-size pieces

• 1 garlic bulb, split into cloves, unpeeled

• 6 bay leaves, stalks removed, finely chopped

• 4 tbsp olive oil

• zest and juice 1 lemon

Instructions

• STEP 1

Heat oven to 200C/180C fan/gas 6. Place the cauliflower, garlic and bay leaves in a large bowl, toss with the oil, zest and juice and season generously. Spread evenly onto a baking sheet (use 2 if you need to). Roast for 20 mins, turning halfway, until al dente and caramelised.

Harissa-crumbed fish with lentils & peppers

Ingredients

• 2 x 200g pouches cooked puy lentils

• 200g jar roasted red peppers, drained and torn into chunks

• 50g black olives, from a jar, roughly chopped

- 1 lemon, zested and cut into wedges

- 3 tbsp olive or rapeseed oil

- 4 x 140g cod fillets (or another white fish)

- 100g fresh breadcrumbs

- 1 tbsp harissa

- ½ small pack flat-leaf parsley, chopped

Instructions

- STEP 1

Heat oven to 200C/180C fan/gas 6. Mix the lentils, peppers, olives, lemon zest, 2 tbsp oil and some seasoning in a roasting tin. Top with the fish fillets. Mix the breadcrumbs, harissa and the remaining oil and put a few spoonfuls on top of each piece of fish. Bake for 12-15 mins until the fish is cooked, the topping is crispy and the lentils are hot. Scatter with the parsley and squeeze over the lemon wedges.

Spinach & courgette lasagne

Ingredients

• 400g spinach

• 1 tbsp olive oil

• 2 garlic cloves, crushed

• 250g mascarpone

• 1 tsp ground nutmeg

• 100g parmesan (or vegetarian alternative), grated

• 9 lasagne sheets

• 100ml double cream

• 3 large courgettes, sliced lengthways

Instructions

• STEP 1

Pour boiling water over the spinach in a sieve or colander to wilt it. Leave until cool enough to handle, then squeeze out any excess liquid. Heat the oil in a non-stick frying pan over a medium heat, add the garlic and soften for 1 min. Tip in the nutmeg and cook for 1 min more, then add the mascarpone, spinach, half the cream and half the parmesan. Season generously, stir well and set aside.

• STEP 2

Heat oven to 180C/160C fan/gas 4. Spread a third of the filling over the base of a 20 x 30cm baking dish, cover with 3 lasagne sheets, then add a layer of courgettes. Repeat twice more. Pour the remaining cream over the final layer and sprinkle over the remaining parmesan. Bake for 40-45 mins or until the sauce is bubbling and the pasta has no resistance when you push a skewer through. Rest for 5 mins, then serve.

Zesty haddock with crushed potatoes & peas

Ingredients

- 600g floury potato, unpeeled, cut into chunks

- 140g frozen peas

- 2 ½ tbsp extra-virgin olive oil

- juice and zest ½ lemon

- 1 tbsp capers, roughly chopped

- 2 tbsp snipped chives

• 4 haddock or other chunky white fish fillets, about 120g each (or use 2 small per person)

• 2 tbsp plain flour

• broccoli, to serve

Instructions

• STEP 1

Cover the potatoes in cold water, bring to the boil, then turn to a simmer. Cook for 10 mins until tender, adding peas for the final min of cooking. Drain and roughly crush together, adding plenty of seasoning and 1 tbsp oil. Keep warm.

• STEP 2

Meanwhile, for the dressing, mix 1 tbsp oil, the lemon juice and zest, capers and chives with some seasoning.

• STEP 3

Dust the fish in the flour, tapping off any excess and season. Heat remaining oil in a non-stick frying pan. Fry the fish for 2-3 mins on each side until cooked, then add the dressing and warm through. Serve with the crush and broccoli.

SNACKS AND SHAKES: HIGH-CALORIE OPTIONS BETWEEN MEALS

Gooseberry & almond streusel squares

Ingredients

- 250g chilled butter, chopped

- 250g self-raising flour

- 125g ground almonds

- 125g light muscovado sugar

- 350g gooseberries, fresh or frozen

- 85g caster sugar, plus extra

- 50g flaked almonds

Instructions

• STEP 1

Heat oven to 190C/170C fan/gas 5. Line a 27 x 18cm baking tin with baking parchment.

• STEP 2

Rub the butter into the flour, almonds and sugar to make crumbs, then firmly press two-thirds onto the base and sides of the tin. Toss the gooseberries with the caster sugar, then scatter over the top.

• STEP 3

Mix the flaked almonds into the remaining crumbs, then scatter over the gooseberries. Bake for 50 mins-1 hr until golden and the fruit is bubbling a little around the edges. Dredge with caster sugar, then cool in the tin. Cut into about 8 squares and enjoy with a cup of tea or serve as a pudding with custard or cream.

Cheese, apple & potato pasties

Ingredients

• 300g cold butter

• 500g plain flour, plus extra for dusting

• 2 medium potatoes (about 400g), halved and thinly sliced

• 3 Granny Smith apples, peeled and sliced

• 350g hard cheese, grated (Lincolnshire Poacher or Cornish cheddar work well)

Instructions

• STEP 1

Line a baking tray with baking parchment. Dice 250g of the butter and tip into a mixing bowl. Add the flour,

1 tsp salt and 1½ tsp black pepper and rub together with your fingers until the mixture resembles fine breadcrumbs, or use a food processor. Stir in 8 tbsp cold water, then bring the mixture together with your hands to create a firm, smooth dough. Cover and chill for 20 mins.

• STEP 2

Cut the dough into six equal-sized pieces and roll each portion into a ball. Chill, covered, for a further 15 mins. Meanwhile, tip the potatoes, apples, cheese and some seasoning into a bowl and toss together.

• STEP 3

Lightly dust a work surface with flour, then roll out one of the dough balls to form a 22cm round. Spoon one-sixth of the potato mix down the centre of the round, then pinch the edges together to make a sealed parcel. Repeat with the remaining dough balls and filling.

Transfer the pasties to the lined baking tray and chill for 30 mins.

• STEP 4

Heat the oven to 220C/200Cfan/gas7. Melt the remaining butter in a small saucepan over a low heat, then generously brush over the pasties. Bake for 20 mins, then turn the heat down to 200C/180C fan/gas 6 and cook for 25-30 mins more, or until golden brown.

Courgette & feta muffins

Ingredients

• 200g self-raising flour

• 1 tsp baking powder

• ½ tsp bicarbonate of soda

• ½ tsp cumin seeds

* 1 large egg

* 150ml buttermilk

* 5 tbsp sunflower oil

* 1 small courgette (about 140g/5oz) grated and squeezed to remove any liquid

* 100g feta, crumbled

Instructions

* STEP 1

Heat oven to 200C/180C fan/gas 6 and line 9 holes of a muffin tray with paper cases. In a bowl, combine the flour, baking powder, bicarbonate of soda, cumin and 1/4 tsp salt.

* STEP 2

In a jug, whisk together the egg, buttermilk and oil. Pour the wet Ingredients into the dry, and add the courgette and half the feta. Stir to just combine, but don't overmix.

• STEP 3

Divide the mixture between the muffin cases, and top with the remaining feta. Bake for 18-20 mins until golden brown. A skewer inserted to the centre of a muffin should come out clean and dry when the muffins are cooked. Cool on a wire rack. Will keep for 2 days in an airtight container.

Cheese & pickle pinwheels

Ingredients

• 100g strong cheddar, grated

• 50g Lancashire cheese, grated

* 2 heaped tbsp pickle

* 1 tsp English mustard powder

* 320g sheet all-butter puff pastry

* 1 beaten egg

Instructions

* STEP 1

Heat the oven to 200C/180C fan/gas 6. Mix the cheeses together. Mix through the pickle and English mustard powder. Unravel the pastry on a lightly floured surface, spread the cheese mixture over and tightly roll into a sausage shape from the longest side. Trim off the ends. Cut into 10 rounds and put on a lined baking sheet (swirl-side up), brush with the egg and bake for 15-20 mins or until golden brown. Leave to cool a little before eating.

Nutty chocolate crunch

Ingredients

• 250g assorted biscuits, roughly chopped

• 250g assorted nuts, or a mix of nuts and dried fruit

• 300g milk or plain chocolate, or a mixture of both, chopped

• 100g butter, chopped

• 140g golden syrup

Instructions

• STEP 1

Butter and line a 20cm square tin with non-stick baking parchment. In a large bowl, combine the biscuits and nuts, halving any larger nuts. Melt the chocolate, butter and golden syrup in a bowl set over a pan of simmering water, stirring occasionally until smooth and glossy, then pour this over the biscuit and nut mixture.

• STEP 2

Tip the mixture into the tin, then flatten lightly – it doesn't need to be completely smooth. Chill for at least 2 hrs or overnight before cutting into squares.

Double ginger cookies

Ingredients

• 350g plain flour

• 1 tbsp ground ginger

• 1 tsp bicarbonate of soda

• 175g light muscovado sugar

• 100g butter, chopped

• 8 pieces of stem ginger, chopped (not too finely), plus thin slices, to decorate (optional)

• 1 large egg

• 4 tbsp golden syrup

• 200g bar dark chocolate, chopped

Instructions

• STEP 1

Mix the flour, ground ginger, bicarbonate of soda, 1/2 tsp salt and sugar in a bowl, then rub in the butter to make crumbs. Stir in the chopped stem ginger.

• STEP 2

Beat together the egg and syrup, pour into the dry Ingredients and stir, then knead with your hands to make a dough. Cut the dough in half and shape each piece into a thick sausage about 6cm across, making sure that the ends are straight. Wrap in cling film and chill for 20 mins. You can now freeze all or part of the dough for 2 months.

• STEP 3

Heat oven to 180C/160C fan/gas 4 and line 2 baking sheets with baking parchment. Thickly slice each sausage into 12 and put the slices on the baking sheets, spacing them well apart and reshaping any, if necessary, to make rounds. Bake for 12 mins, then leave to cool for a few mins to harden before transferring to a wire rack to cool completely.

• STEP 4

Melt the chocolate in a bowl over a pan of gently simmering water, making sure that the water isn't touching the bottom of the bowl. Dip half of each cookie into the chocolate – you may need to spoon it over when you get to the final few. Decorate with a slice of ginger, if you like, and leave to set. Will keep for 1 week in an airtight container.

Leek, mushroom & gruyère quiche

Ingredients

• 25g butter

• 4 leeks, sliced and washed

• 250g pack chestnut mushroom, sliced

• 2 eggs

• 284ml double cream

• 140g gruyère, coarsely grated

For the pastry

• 280g plain flour

• 140g cold butter, cut into pieces

Instructions

• STEP 1

To make the pastry, tip the flour and butter into a bowl, then rub together with your fingertips until completely mixed and crumbly. Add 8 tbsp cold water, then bring everything together with your hands until just combined. Roll into a ball and use straight away or chill for up to 2 days. The pastry can also be frozen for up to a month.

• STEP 2

Roll out the pastry on a lightly floured surface to a round about 5cm larger than a 25cm tin. Use your rolling pin to lift it up, then drape over the tart case so there is an overhang of pastry on the sides. Using a small ball of pastry scraps, push the pastry into the corners of the tin (see picture, above left). Chill in the fridge or freezer for 20 mins. Heat oven to 200C/fan 180C/gas 6.

• STEP 3

While the pastry is chilling, heat the butter in a pan and cook the leeks for 10 mins, stirring occasionally, until they soften. Then turn up the heat and add the mushrooms. Cook for 5 mins more, then turn off the heat.

• STEP 4

Lightly prick the base of the tart with a fork, line the tart case with a large circle of greaseproof paper or foil, then fill with baking beans. Blind-bake the tart for 20 mins, remove the paper and beans, then continue to cook for 5-10 mins until biscuit brown

• STEP 5

While the tart case cooks, beat the eggs in a bowl, then gradually add the cream. Stir in the leeks, mushrooms and half the cheese. Season, then tip the filling into the tart case. Sprinkle with the rest of the cheese, then bake for 20-25 mins until set and golden brown. Leave to cool in the case, trim the edges of the pastry, then remove and serve in slices.

Layered rainbow salad pots

Ingredients

• 350g pasta shapes (De Cecco is a good brand that stays nice and firm)

• 200g green beans, trimmed and chopped into short lengths

• 160g can tuna in olive oil, drained

* 4 tbsp mayonnaise

* 4 tbsp natural yogurt

* ½ small pack chives, snipped (optional)

* 200g cherry tomatoes, quartered

* 1 orange pepper, cut into little cubes 195g can sweetcorn, drained

Instructions

* STEP 1

Cook the pasta until it is still a little al dente (2 mins less than the pack instructions) and drain well. Cook the green beans in simmering water for 2 mins, then rinse in cold water and drain well. Mix the tuna with the mayonnaise and yogurt. Add the chives, if using.

* STEP 2

Tip the pasta into a large glass bowl or four small ones, or four wide-necked jars (useful for taking on picnics). Spoon the tuna dressing over the top of the pasta. Add a layer of green beans, followed by a layer of cherry tomatoes, then the pepper and sweetcorn. Cover and chill until you're ready to eat.

Smoked paprika prawn skewers

Ingredients

• 12 large raw prawns

• ½ tbsp smoked Spanish paprika (sweet or hot, whichever you prefer)

• 2 large garlic cloves, finely chopped

• 1 tsp cumin seeds, toased and ground

• couple of oregano sprigs, leaves finely chopped, or ½ tsp dried

• juice and zest of 1 large lemon

• 2 tbsp olive oil

You will also need:

• 12 mini wooden skewers

Instructions

• STEP 1

Soak the skewers in a bowl of water for 10 mins. Meanwhile, peel the prawns, leaving the tails intact, and devein. To do this, run a sharp knife down the back, making a tiny incision just enough to remove the visible black vein. Wash the prawns and pat dry with kitchen paper.

• STEP 2

In a medium-sized bowl, mix together the paprika, garlic, cumin, oregano, lemon zest and 1 tbsp olive oil. Add the prawns and leave to marinate for 15 mins at room temperature. Then skewer a prawn onto each stick.

• STEP 3

Heat the remaining oil in a roomy frying pan and fry the prawns for 3-4 mins, turning halfway through until just cooked. You may need to do this in batches. Season, squeeze over some lemon juice and serve.

Carrot cake fridge flapjacks

Ingredients

• 170g butter, chopped, plus extra for the tin

• 200g pitted dates, roughly chopped

• 250g honey

- 2 large carrots, coarsely grated

- 300g rolled oats

- 100g dried cranberries

- 150g dried apricots, chopped

- 70g chopped walnuts

- 70g mixed seeds

- 2 tsp mixed spice

- 2 tsp ground cinnamon

For the icing

- 1 tbsp soft cheese

- 2 tbsp icing sugar, sieved

- 1 small orange, zested, plus 1-2 tbsp orange juice

Instructions

• STEP 1

Boil the kettle. Heat the oven to 170C/150C fan/gas 3½, butter a 20 x 30cm cake tin and line with baking parchment. Tip the dates into a heatproof bowl and cover with 60ml boiling water from the kettle. Set aside to rehydrate for 10 mins, then tip into a food processor and blitz until smooth.

• STEP 2

Melt the butter and honey in a saucepan over a low heat, stirring until smooth. Tip the carrots, oats, cranberries, apricots, chopped walnuts, mixed seeds, mixed spice, cinnamon and a small pinch of salt into a large bowl. Stir the sweetened butter and puréed dates into the dry Ingredients until combined, then tip into the prepared tin and press into an even layer using a spatula. Bake for 45-50 mins, covering with foil halfway through if the flapjacks brown too quickly.

Cool in the tin. Once completely cool, chill in the fridge for at least 3 hrs.

• STEP 3

For the icing, whisk all of the Ingredients together until smooth. Drizzle the icing over the flapjacks and cut into 12 bars. Will keep, covered in the fridge, for three days.

Buckwheat galettes

Ingredients

• 80g buckwheat flour

• 5 medium eggs

• 250ml milk

• 2 tsp Dijon mustard

• 4 tbsp single cream

• 100g mature gruyère, comté or cheddar, grated

• butter, for frying

• 100g ham, torn

• fried mushrooms or steamed spinach, to serve (optional)

Instructions

• STEP 1

Mix the flour, 1 egg, the milk and a pinch of salt in a jug or bowl. Set aside for 30 mins, or up to 3 hrs. Mash together the mustard, cream and cheese in another bowl. Heat the oven to 200C/180C fan/gas 6, and line two baking trays with baking parchment or foil.

• STEP 2

Melt the butter in a large frying pan, then once foaming, add enough batter to just cover the pan, swirling it to cover the surface in a thin layer (pour any excess back into the batter bowl). Cook until the surface is set and the underside is browning, carefully flip and cook for another minute or 2, then take off the heat.

• STEP 3

Spoon a quarter of the cheese mixture onto the middle of the pancake, using the spoon to create space in the centre to hold an egg. Crack one into the space and lay a few pieces of ham around the edges. Fold each side of the pancake in towards the centre to make a square. Cook in the pan for another 30 secs-1 min, then transfer to a baking tray. Repeat with the rest of the pancakes, then bake for 6-7 mins until the egg whites are set. Serve with fried mushrooms or wilted spinach, if you like.

Apple 'doughnuts'

Ingredients

- 150g soft cheese

- 2 tsp honey

- 3 apples (use a crunchy eating variety)

- 3-4 tbsp almond or peanut butter (optional)

- coloured sprinkles, to decorate

Instructions

- STEP 1

Mix the soft cheese with the honey and set aside. Peel the apples, then slice each through the core into five or six rings, about 1cm thick. Use an apple corer or small round biscuit cutter to stamp out a circle from the middle of each slice, removing the core and creating 'doughnut' shapes. Pat the slices dry using kitchen paper – they should be as dry as possible to help the toppings stick.

• STEP 2

Spread some nut butter over the slices, if using, then top with the sweetened soft cheese. Decorate with the sprinkles and serve.

Spicy plum & apple chutney

Ingredients

• 1 garlic bulb

• thumb-size piece fresh root ginger

• 2 large onions

• 1kg Bramley apples

- 3 star anise

- 1 tsp cumin seed

- 1 cinnamon stick

- 500ml bottle cider vinegar

- 1 tbsp salt

- 1kg plums

- 450g golden caster sugar

You will also need

- 4-5 sterilised jars

Instructions

- STEP 1

To sterilise the jars: run them with the lids and any rubber seals through the hottest cycle of your dishwasher. If you don't have a dishwasher, give the jars a good wash, then heat them in the oven at 150C/130C fan/ gas 2 for 30 mins. Don't bake seals – boil them in a pan of water for 10 mins. If you don't have lids you can buy jam pot covers from cook shops which you can then cover with fabric.

• STEP 2

Prepare the Ingredients: first, peel the garlic cloves and cut them into slivers. Peel and thinly shred the ginger. Halve, peel and thinly slice the onions, then put them in a large, wide saucepan or a preserving pan with the garlic and ginger. Peel, core and chop the apples, then add to the pan with the spices, vinegar and salt.

• STEP 3

Bring the pan to the boil over a gentle heat, give everything a good stir, then turn down the heat and cover the pan (if you don't have a lid use foil). Simmer for 30 mins until the apples are cooked and pulpy.

• STEP 4

While the apples are simmering, stone and quarter the plums, then add them to the cooked apples with the sugar. Stir well and leave to bubble away, this time uncovered, for another 40 mins stirring regularly until the plums are cooked but still retain some of their shape. Ladle into the sterilised jars, seal and label.

• STEP 5

This chutney is best kept for about a month before eating as the vinegar needs a bit of time to mellow. If you don't want the flavour of the spices to develop any more, then take out the cinnamon and star anise before potting. It will keep for 1 year in a cool place but once opened store in the fridge and use within a month.

Smoked mackerel risotto

Ingredients

- 1 tbsp butter

- 1 onion, finely chopped

- 250g risotto rice

- 100ml white wine

- 1l vegetable stock

- 1 x 240 pack smoked mackerel

- 2 spring onions, sliced

- 100g bag fresh spinach

Instructions

• STEP 1

Heat the butter in a large frying pan. Tip in the onion, then fry gently for 5 mins until softened. Stir in the rice and mix until coated in the butter, then pour in the wine and let it bubble until it's almost all disappeared.

• STEP 2

Pour in half the stock, give it a good stir, then leave to gently cook for 10 mins. Add half of the remaining stock, stir again and cook for 5 mins more. Keep adding stock and cooking until the rice is tender.

• STEP 3

Peel the skin off the mackerel, scrape away any dark brown flesh, then flake. Stir into the rice with the spring onions and spinach, then cook just until the spinach has wilted slightly. Serve straight away.

Flat apple & vanilla tart

Ingredients

- 375g pack puff pastry, preferably all-butter

- 5 large eating apples - Cox's, russets or Elstar

- juice of 1 lemon

- 25g butter, cut into small pieces

- 3 tsp vanilla sugar or 1 tsp vanilla extract

- 1 tbsp caster sugar

- 3 rounded tbsp apricot conserve

Instructions

- STEP 1

Heat oven to 220C/fan 200C/gas 7. Roll out the pastry and trim to a round about 35cm across. Transfer to a baking sheet lined with parchment paper.

• STEP 2

Peel, core and thinly slice the apples and toss in the lemon juice. Spread over the pastry to within 2cm of the edges. Curl up the edges slightly to stop the juices running off.

• STEP 3

Dot the top with the butter and sprinkle with vanilla and caster sugar. Bake for 15-20 mins until the apples are tender and the pastry crisp.

• STEP 4

Warm the conserve and brush over the apples and pastry edge. Serve hot with vanilla ice cream or crème fraîche.

White chocolate & raspberry flapjacks

Ingredients

- 200g unsalted butter

- 200g demerara sugar

- 200g honey or golden syrup

- 400g oats

- 200g white chocolate chips

- 20g freeze-dried raspberries

For the topping

- 250g white chocolate

- 150g fresh raspberries

- 10g freeze-dried raspberries

Instructions

- STEP 1

Heat the oven to 180C/160C fan/gas 4 and line a 23 x 23cm square baking tin with baking parchment. Tip the butter, sugar and honey into a medium pan over a low-medium heat, and stir until everything has melted together.

- STEP 2

Tip the oats into a large bowl, then pour over the buttery sugar mixture and stir to combine. Leave to cool for 5 mins, then fold in the white chocolate chips and freeze-dried raspberries. Tip the flapjack mix into the prepared tin and press into the base. Bake for 20-24 mins until golden and crisp at the edges. Leave to cool in the tin for 2 hrs.

• STEP 3

For the topping, melt the white chocolate in a heatproof bowl set over a pan of simmering water, ensuring the bowl doesn't touch the water, or in 20-second bursts in the microwave. Pour this over the cooled flapjacks, spread to the edges, then scatter over the fresh and freeze-dried raspberries. Leave to set for 1 hr, then cut into 12 large or 24 small squares. Will keep chilled for three days. Serve at room temperature.

Banana cake

Ingredients

• 100g softened unsalted butter

• 140g light muscovado sugar

• 2 large eggs

• 3 large ripe bananas, mashed (about 450g/1lb total weight)

• 50g pecans, roughly chopped

• 50g raisins

• 150ml buttermilk

• 280g plain flour

• 1 tsp bicarbonate of soda

• 50g icing sugar

Instructions

• STEP 1

Preheat the oven to fan 160C/ conventional 180C/gas 4. Butter a 20 x 13cm loaf tin and line the base with greaseproof paper.

• STEP 2

In a large bowl, whisk together the butter and sugar with an electric whisk until creamy. Beat in the eggs one at a time (don't worry that the mixture looks curdled). Stir in the mashed bananas, pecans, raisins and buttermilk.

• STEP 3

Sift the flour and bicarbonate of soda on top of the banana mixture, then fold in until evenly mixed, taking care not to overmix. Spoon into the prepared tin and level the top.

• STEP 4

Bake for 1 hour 15 minutes until a skewer pushed in the centre comes out almost, but not quite, dry. Remove from the oven and leave for about 10 minutes, then turn it out of the tin on to a cooling rack to cool.

- STEP 5

For the icing, mix the icing sugar with 2-3 tsp cold water to give a smooth, runny consistency. Using a dessertspoon, drizzle the icing in lines across the loaf.

Crisp chicken bites

Ingredients

- 4 boneless chicken breast fillets

- 6 tbsp red pesto

- 3 large handfuls breadcrumbs, frsh or dried (about 300g/10oz)

- olive oil

Instructions

- STEP 1

Cut the chicken breasts into small chunks, each about the size of a marble (you should get roughly 15 pieces per breast). Put the pesto in a bowl and mix together with the chicken until coated all over. Tip the breadcrumbs into a large freezer bag.

• STEP 2

Add the chicken pieces in batches to the bag and give it a good shake to coat. Place a piece of greaseproof paper on a baking sheet, then lay the chicken pieces on the sheet, making sure none of them are touching. Put in the freezer and, when frozen solid, take off the baking sheet and store in a container or freezer bag.

• STEP 3

To cook, heat oven to 220C/fan 200C/ gas 7. Pour a little oil onto a shallow baking tray, just enough to cover it. Put the tray in the oven and let it heat up for 5 mins. Tip the chicken onto the sheet and return to the oven for 10-15 mins until crisp and cooked through.

Marshmallows dipped in chocolate

Ingredients

• 50g white chocolate

• 50g milk chocolate

• selection of cake sprinkles

• 1 bag marshmallows (about 200g)

• 1 pack lollipop sticks

Instructions

• STEP 1

Heat the chocolate in separate bowls over simmering water or on a low setting in the microwave. Allow to cool a little.

• STEP 2

Put your chosen sprinkles on separate plates. Push a cake pop or lolly stick into a marshmallow about half way in. Dip into the white or milk chocolate, allow the excess to drip off then dip into the sprinkles of your choice. Put into a tall glass to set. Repeat with each marshmallow.

Passion fruit curd

Ingredients

• 200g/7oz passion fruit pulp, about 6-8 ripe passion fruits

• 3 large eggs

• 140g butter, diced

• 250g golden caster sugar

• 2 tsp cornflour

Instructions

• STEP 1

Put the passion fruit pulp in a food processor and whizz to separate the seeds from all the juicy bits. Scrape into a sieve set over a medium saucepan, pushing through as much pulp as you can. Reserve 2 tbsp of the seeds, then discard the rest.

• STEP 2

Add the remaining Ingredients to the pan and set over a low heat. Whisk until all the butter has melted then, using a wooden spoon, stir constantly until the passion fruit curd has thickened to a similar consistency as lemon curd. Don't be tempted to turn the heat up to speed up the process as the eggs will curdle; make sure you stir right around the edge, too, as this is where it might catch first.

• STEP 3

Sieve the curd into a clean bowl to get rid of any eggy bits that may have curdled. Stir in the reserved seeds and cool, before spooning into jars and chilling. Curd will keep in the fridge for a week. Eat smothered on hot buttered toast, crumpets or scones.

SECTION V: FINALLY!

Incorporating Resistance Training for Muscle Growth

If your goal is to gain weight and increase your muscle mass, combining nutrition with intentional exercise is important.

Combine your dietary efforts with a structured strength or resistance training program. This can help promote muscle growth and ensure that the weight you gain is lean muscle mass. Strength training helps break down muscle fibers and repair and rebuild them stronger and larger over time.

Strength training equipment can include dumbbells, weight machines, kettlebells, resistance bands, and medicine balls. You can even use your body weight if you're just getting started or don't have equipment.

Examples of strength training exercises include:

• Abdominal exercises

• Bench press

• Curls

• Kettlebell swings

• Leg lifts

• Leg press

• Shoulder press

• Squats

• Tricep extensions

Regularly engaging in a strength training regimen requires additional protein and calories in your diet plan. This ensures that you're getting enough to prevent weight loss and support new muscle growth. If you have questions about properly fueling your workouts for optimal muscle mass gain, working with a registered dietitian to devise a meal plan is helpful.

Safety and Well-Being: Tips for Reaching Your Weight Gain Goal

Weight gain, just like weight loss, should be a gradual process. Anything that promises instant results isn't designed to set you up for long-term success or sustainability. When embarking on a weight gain journey, keep safety and well-being in mind with the following tips:

• **Consult a healthcare professional**: Before making significant changes to your diet, consult a healthcare provider, like a registered dietitian. They can assess your individual health needs and provide personalized guidance.

• **Make gradual changes:** Avoid making quick and drastic changes to your diet. Gradually increase your calorie intake to allow your body to adjust and minimize the risk of digestive issues.

• **Stay hydrated:** Adequate hydration is crucial for overall health. Drink plenty of water throughout the day to support digestion and prevent dehydration.

• **Limit ultra-processed foods:** Though increasing calorie intake is essential, avoid relying on unhealthy, ultra-processed foods that are high in saturated fats and sugars, which don't benefit your health. Instead, opt for whole, minimally processed foods that can help promote weight gain while supporting overall well-being.

• **Track your progress:** Monitor your weight gain and adjust your diet and activity routines accordingly. If you're not gaining weight as expected, consult a healthcare provider to identify any underlying issues.

Finally, Gaining weight can be a complex and challenging process for individuals. Understanding and addressing the potential challenges can help individuals navigate the journey more effectively. By addressing factors such as metabolism, appetite, dietary restrictions, lifestyle, medical conditions, psychological factors, and seeking appropriate knowledge and guidance, individuals can overcome these challenges and achieve their weight gain goals.